QUICK & EASY stress busters

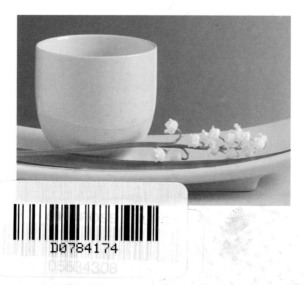

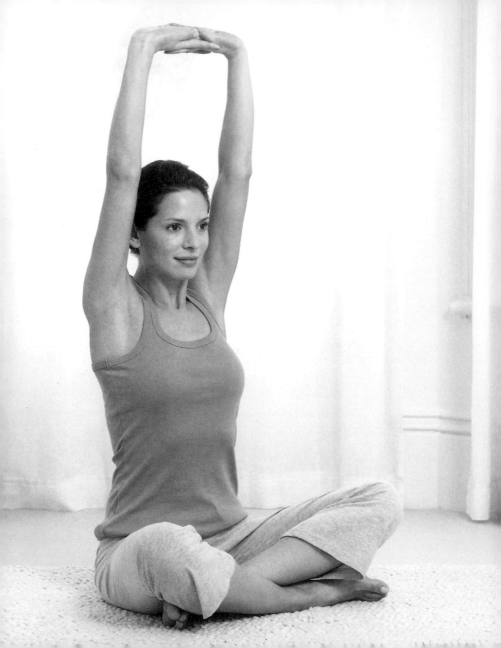

DUNCAN BAIRD PUBLISHERS
LONDON

QUICK & EASY stress busters

Anna Selby

5-minute routines for

anyone

anytime

anywhere

QUICK & EASY stress busters

Anna Selby

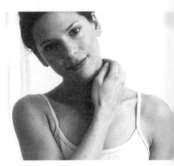

First published in the United Kingdom and Ireland in 2009 by
Duncan Baird Publishers Ltd
Sixth Floor
Castle House
75–76 Wells Street
London WIT 3QH

Conceived, created and designed by Duncan Baird Publishers

Managing Editor: Grace Cheetham
Editors: Joanna Micklem and Zoë Fargher
Managing Designer: Manisha Patel
Designer: Jantje Doughty
Commissioned photography: Jules Selmes

British Library Cataloguing-in-Publication Data:
A CIP record for this book is available from the British Library

ISBN: 978-1-84483-783-0

10 9 8 7 6 5 4 3 2 1

Typeset in Gill Sans, Nofret and Helvetica Neue
Colour reproduction by Scanhouse, Malaysia
Printed in China by Imago

Publisher's notes: The information in this book is not intended as a
substitute for professional medical advice and treatment. If you are
pregnant or are suffering from any medical conditions or health problems,
it is recommended that you consult a medical professional before
following any of the advice or practice suggested in this book. Duncan
Baird Publishers, or any other persons who have been involved in
working on this publication, cannot accept responsibility for any injuries
or damage incurred as a result of following the information, exercises or
therapeutic techniques contained in this book.

contents

introduction

Think of the excitement of playing a competitive sport, the challenge of learning a new skill, the exhilaration of an adventurous trip. These are all examples of stressful situations – but remove them, and life would be pretty dull. We tend to think of stress as negative, and forget that a certain level of stress can stimulate us into action – we need some stress in our lives, and it may even be good for us! However, these forms of "good" stress all have one thing in common: a finite goal. We anticipate something, get excited and wound up, the situation happens (whether it's a party, a sports game or an exam), then it's over, and we can calm down and move on with our lives.

Problems arise when stressful situations, and our reactions to them, become chronic. The human body has not changed fundamentally since prehistory, when stress usually meant mortal danger, requiring an instant physical response of "fight or flight". Our bodies still respond to stress the same way today: the adrenal glands release the hormone adrenalin (epinephrine), while the sympathetic nervous system goes into overdrive, diverting blood to your heart and skeletal muscles, and away from body systems you wouldn't need while you were fighting or fleeing, such as your skin and digestion.

In the short-term, these physical reactions are not harmful. However, daily strains including uncomfortable commuting, feeling overly pressured at work, nagging financial anxieties or life-changing emotional turmoil can contribute to a constant level of stress, and we find ourselves in a vicious circle – while mental and emotional stress affects our body, physical stress impacts on our mind. Physical symptoms of excessive stress include headaches, skin eruptions or digestive disorders, while mental and emotional ones can range from insomnia and exhaustion to feelings of anger, impotence and depression.

tackling stress

So if you want to address your reactions to stress, what can you do? There are two basic approaches: exercise and relaxation. If your body is charged with adrenalin from a stressful situation, exercise provides a physical outlet. In addition, strenuous exercise produces endorphins, the body's natural opiates, giving you a temporary "high". Exercise will also relieve mental and emotional stress, because while you are exercising your mind will be focused on and involved in your body's activity.

Through the use of relaxation techniques, you can prevent stress from becoming damaging by inducing a state of physical and mental calm. The techniques can include movement as well as stationary meditation, because when either the mind or the body relaxes, the other naturally follows suit. Sometimes, just by relaxing your body, you

7

will find that your energy seems to be revitalized. In turn, this renewed flow of energy will boost your body's strength, and even your immune system – making you feel fitter and more confident.

how to use this book

I've covered a wide range of exercise, meditation and bodywork techniques in this book, but each exercise is simple and quick enough to use whenever you feel under pressure. Scan through the book, and if something catches your eye, try it out. I have organized the first two chapters into exercises for particular times of day and situations. Chapter three tackles stress in specific areas of the body, while chapter four gives you options for when you need to lift your mood. Chapter five offers techniques for de-stressing with a partner. If you have more time, or you want to take your relaxation to a deeper level, you can build the exercises up into a sequence, as I've explained on pages 124–5. Here is a quick introduction to each discipline you'll find in this book, and there is some general advice on practising them on pages 16–19.

chi gung

The healing system known as chi gung (also written as chi kung or qigong) originated in China more than 2,000 years ago. Chi gung

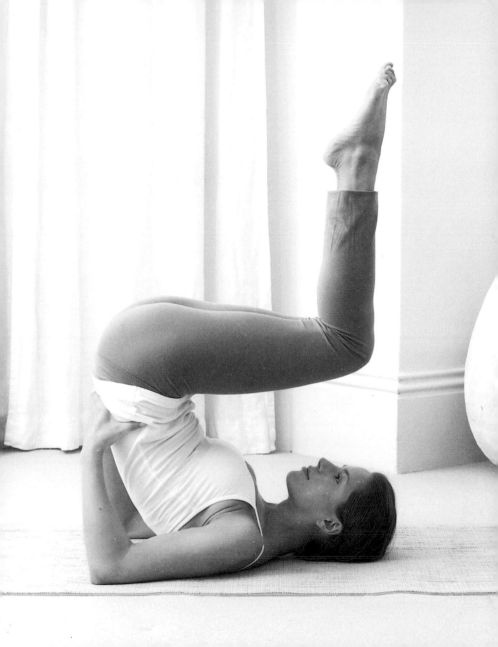

exercises are based on the concept of chi, the flow of universal energy that, according to Chinese medicine, courses through everything from the stars to the humblest ant. Chi flows through the body in a network of meridians, not dissimilar to the nervous or circulatory system, and it is our life force, animating our bodies and minds. When our chi flows freely, we are in harmony, but when it is blocked, and the flow of chi is interrupted, we lose vitality. Chi gung techniques promote the flow of chi and are both restorative and relaxing. If you have a few minutes before you begin practising chi gung, close your eyes and take five deep, relaxed breaths. Maintain this breathing as you practise.

massage

You may think of massage as the ultimate luxury, to be performed with scented oils by a sensitive practitioner in beautiful surroundings. In reality, anyone can learn to massage, and it is one of the simplest and most effective ways to alleviate stress, calming the mind and releasing and relieving tense muscles. Most of the massages in this book are quick self-massages, which you can adapt to almost any situation. They target key areas where we all store tension, such as the shoulders, neck and face, and I've drawn from a number of massage types, including shiatsu, reflexology and aromatherapy. Massage is also a wonderfully

10

relaxing thing to share with your partner or a friend, and so I have also
included some massages in chapter five.

If you use essential oils in a massage, choose oils that have
uplifting and relaxing qualities. These include lavender, rose, neroli,
ylang-ylang, geranium, jasmine and the citrus oils. Dilute 25 drops of
essential oil in 50 ml (2fl oz) of carrier oil, such as almond or grapeseed.
If you are going to use your oil-blend on your face, reduce the amount
of essential oil by half, unless you are using one of the few essential oils
that can be used directly on the skin, such as lavender or rose. Note
that some essential oils are unsuitable for use during pregnancy.

meditation

The aim of meditation is to train the conscious mind to a state of
stillness and tranquillity, making it a very effective way of coping
with stress. People who meditate regularly see physiological benefits
including lowered blood pressure and improved circulation. Most
meditators also report greater clarity in all their thought processes,
better memory and concentration and an ability to stay calm.

The most important thing to remember when you are learning
to meditate is that the intrusion of thoughts is inevitable. Don't get
upset or self-critical when worries, ideas or lists of things to do enter

11

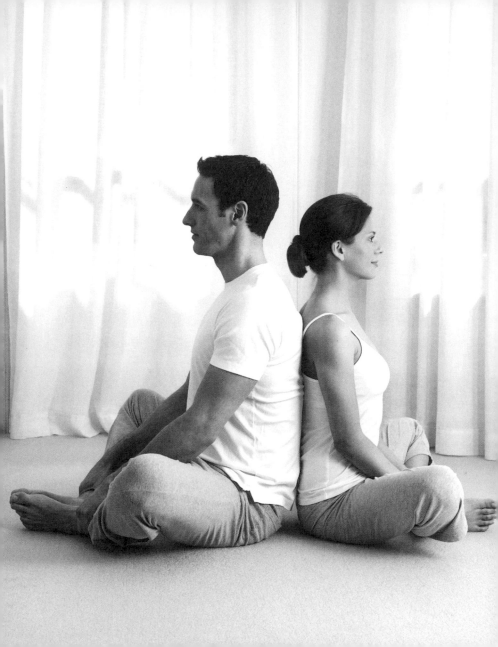

your mind. Observe the stray thought's presence calmly, make no judgement about it, and let it go. Then draw your focus back to your meditation. You don't need to sit in a yoga position, or even on the floor, to meditate – the practice will work just as well if you are sitting in a chair. Just find a quiet spot, make sure you sit with your spine long and straight, and take a few moments to focus on your body and let go of any tensions or worries before you begin.

pilates

Pilates is named after its creator, Joseph Pilates, who developed the technique to combat his own physical frailty, and to help others recuperate from injury. Pilates works on a more subtle, more profound level than many other forms of exercise. If you have ever come out of the gym feeling just as stressed when you went in, one reason may be that if you habitually use a gym machine such as a treadmill, your brain will not be engaged and your mind can wander, often in the direction of what's worrying you. Pilates is sometimes referred to as "thinking exercise", and practising Pilates requires a special synchronicity of mind and body. This results in a sense of wholeness and integration that is more commonly associated with eastern meditation and movement techniques. Concentration is one of the six basic principles of the

13

Pilates system – reflected in Joseph Pilates' own favourite quotation from the poet Schiller, "It is the mind itself that builds the body."

Pilates was first taken up as a rehabilitative technique by dancers, and I have also included some dance movements with the Pilates ones, chosen for their natural ability to relax particular parts of the body or simply because the movements themselves have an uplifting quality.

reiki

Many people think of reiki as a form of massage. It is actually a form of energy work that practitioners believe originated in Tibet before being rediscovered by a Japanese monk in the 19th century. Reiki is a natural healing method that aims to revitalize your life force and balance your body's energies. When giving reiki, you "open" yourself as a channel for universal life energy by mentally relaxing and visualizing the energy passing through your body and into your hands.

Reiki is especially effective in tackling stress-related problems such as headache and lowered immunity. It can also help with pain management, promote mental clarity and lift spirits dulled by anxiety. You can practise reiki as a self-treatment, or with a partner. If you practise with a partner, be aware that it is not the giver's own energy that is transmitted – you should both feel strengthened by the experience.

14

yoga

Yoga postures, or asana, are a renowned antidote to stress. They exercise the whole body, including the internal organs, and because your mental focus stays on your breathing while you practise, your body and mind blend together to form a kind of moving meditation, instilling a deep feeling of tranquillity and calm.

The exercises I've chosen are all simple Hatha yoga poses and sequences. You can also practise some of them dynamically – for example, in Salute to the Sun (see pages 86–9), you can jump rather than step from postion to postion and move continuously rather than holding. I've included a yoga nidra (yogic sleep) meditation on page 36–7. If you have time, practise some yoga poses before this meditation, as this will probably make it easier for you to relax your body and mind.

other techniques

I have drawn inspiration from many other techniques to write this book. Two which I think are worth a brief explanation, are:

• **Autogenic training (AT)** Autogenic means "generated from within", and AT is a relaxation technique that aims to self-empower practitioners so that they can unwind quickly and effectively when necessary. The AT exercise (see page 90–1) in this book outlines

15

four progressive stages. I have adapted the exercise so that you can practise all four stages over the course of a single day (normally they would take several weeks). As you become more adept, you will find that you can use AT as an instant defuser of any stressful situation.

- **Hydrotherapy** A traditional form of naturopathy, hydrotherapy is today much-neglected in the US and UK, although it is still part of mainstream healthcare in continental Europe. Hydrotherapy works by stimulating the body's natural processes through the application of hot and/or cold water. Treatments include baths of numerous kinds, compresses and wraps applied directly to the body, water massages, inhalations and simple movements or exercises performed with the body partially submerged in water. Many people find that the power of water to heal, stimulate and relax is remarkable and profoundly beneficial. Hydrotherapy is particularly effective at strengthening the immune system, which is often adversely affected by stress.

a few suggestions

Here are some general guidelines for practising the various exercises.

- **Clothing** If you are practising Pilates, chi gung or yoga, you may be more comfortable in loose clothing, particularly around your abdominals, as tight waistbands may restrict your breathing.

16

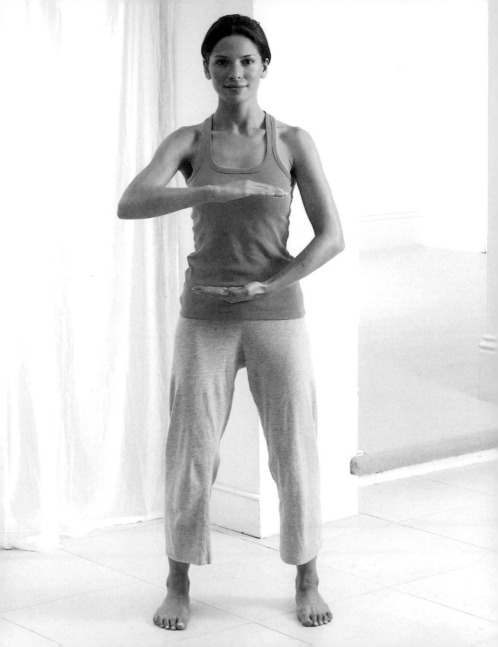

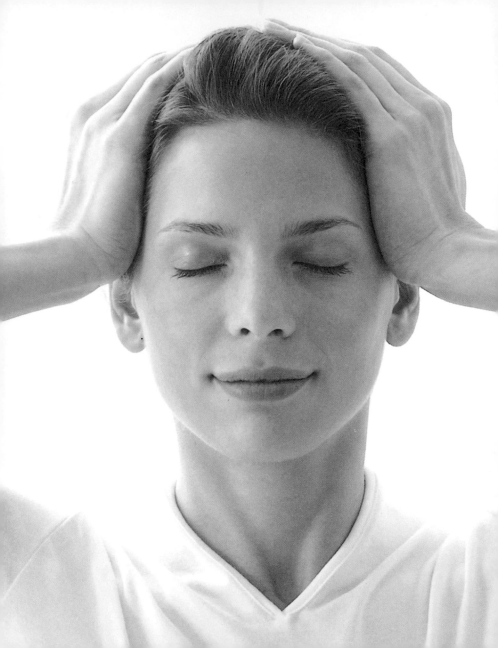

- **Preparation** If you can, find a quiet place in which to practise, so that you don't feel self-conscious or that you might be interrupted. Switch your phone to voicemail, and put your computer to sleep.
- **Space** Before you begin an exercise, read the instructions and check that you have enough space to move freely, if you'll need it. When you are practising standing yoga exercises, it's advisable to use a non-slip surface, such as carpet or a yoga mat.

There are so many ways to relieve stress, and inevitably some will work better for you than others. That's why there's such a diverse range of exercises in this book. So experiment with a number of techniques and be creative with when and where you use them. You don't have to practise the exercise entitled "on your sofa" there – try it out in the bus queue. Similarly, the exercise called "morning meditation" may help to settle your mind before bed. Take note of what you find effective. It may be a dynamic yoga sequence (see pages 86–9), or a slow, calming reiki treatment (see page 50–1). When you find an exercise that works particularly well, make a positive commitment to yourself to practise it every day for week or two. Reducing the harmful effects of stress can make a big difference to your quality of life, physically, mentally and emotionally – and doing so really can be quick and easy.

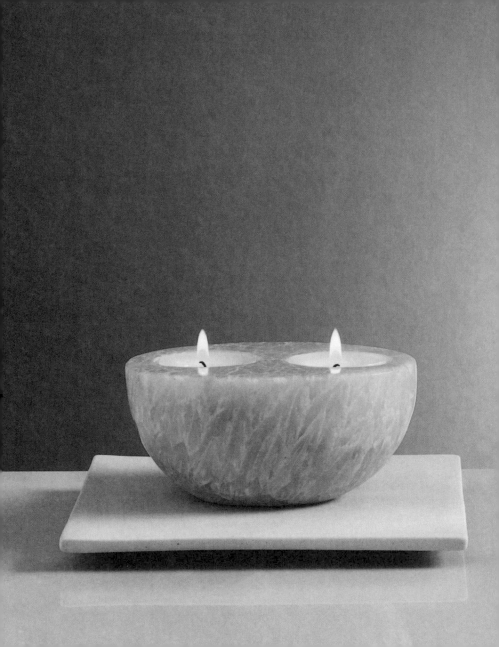

anytime

At different times of day you need to relax for different reasons. This chapter will help you to meet the demands of a working day, and enrich your leisure time. Wake up with an uplifting chi gung exercise, meditate to calm your mind at work, and prepare for a sound night's sleep with massage. You can beat stress and take control – any time.

wake-up stretch
loosening

awaken your body ready for a long, busy day

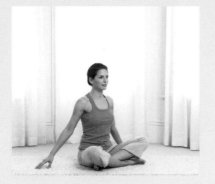 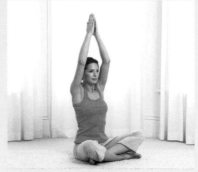

1 Sit on the floor with your legs crossed, back straight and shoulders and neck relaxed. If you are uncomfortable, place a cushion under your hips to lift them slightly. Place your fingertips lightly on the floor about 30cm (1ft) away from your hips. Inhale for five counts, hold your breath for five counts and exhale for five counts.

2 Without moving your shoulders, breathe in and raise your arms, palms facing upward. Press your palms together above your head, keeping your shoulders stable. Feel a stretch from your hips all the way up to your fingertips. Be careful not to push your neck forward. Hold for a count of five and lower your arms. Repeat five times.

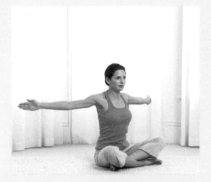 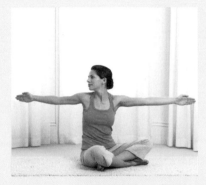

3 Breathe in, lifting your arms in front of you level with your shoulders. Bring your palms together, breathe out, drop your chin to your chest and hold for a count of five. Lift your head and breathe in, opening your arms out to the sides and behind you as you count to five. Breathe out and slowly lower your arms. Repeat five times.

4 Breathe in and lift your arms out to the sides, in line with your shoulders. Breathe out and twist to the right. Twist from your hips, turning your entire upper body, and look toward your right hand. Hold for a count of five as you breathe out. Inhale and come back to the middle, then repeat the twist to your left. Repeat five times.

wake-up stretch

(continued)

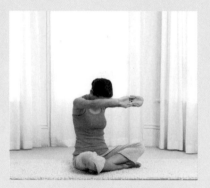
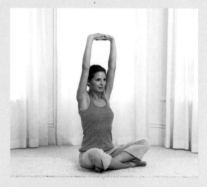

5 Relax your arms and link your fingers together. Breathe in and, without raising your shoulders, stretch your arms straight out in front of you, rotating your wrists so that your palms face away from your shoulders. Now, drop your chin down to your chest and breathe out slowly, elongating the muscles at the back of your neck.

6 Breathe in and lift your head and arms, taking your hands directly above your head. Keep your shoulders stable. Feel the stretch all the way through your body. Hold this position as you count to five. Breathe out, lower your arms and drop your chin to your chest as in step 5. Alternate between these two positions five times.

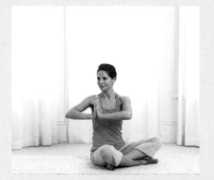

7 Place your hands in prayer position, palms together level with your breastbone, fingers pointing up, forearms parallel to the floor. Breathe in and twist your whole body to the right, keeping your nose in line with your hands. Hold for a count of five, then exhale. Breathe in and twist to the left. Repeat three times on each side.

8 Lower your arms and place your fingertips back on the floor. Check your posture: your spine should be long and straight, and your neck, shoulders and hips should be completely relaxed. Breathe in slowly for five counts, hold for five counts and breathe out for five counts. Repeat this breathing pattern three times.

25

morning
meditation
settling

prepare your mind for the
day ahead with meditation

1 Sit in a comfortable position either on the floor, a chair or a sofa. If you are on the floor, sit with your legs crossed and your back against a wall. If you are on a chair or sofa, place your feet flat on the floor and make sure your back is straight. Rest your hands loosely in your lap and relax your face, neck and shoulders.

2 Before you begin your meditation, take some slow, deep breaths and focus on releasing any areas of tension. Allow any thoughts or worries to surface. Recognize that you will have to deal with these and then put them aside to address later. Notice any tense areas in your body, and relax them as you exhale.

3 Close your eyes and become aware of your breathing. Start to count your breaths: inhale on one, exhale on two, inhale on three and so on. Keep your breathing steady and deep. As you count, bring your attention either to the sensation of air passing through your nose or to the rise and fall of your abdomen.

4 When you lose count – and it's inevitable that you will – simply start counting again. When stray thoughts enter your mind, acknowledge them, put them aside, and return to focusing on your breath as before. Count your breaths for five minutes, then slowly open your eyes, inhale deeply and stretch your body.

27

lunchtime activator
focusing

refresh your outlook with a graceful chi gung exercise

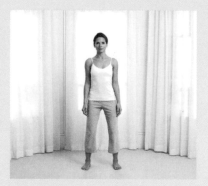 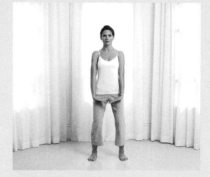

1 Stand with your feet shoulder-width apart, knees slightly bent, arms relaxed down by your sides. Check that your spine is long and straight, and tilt your pelvis forward a little to flatten your lower back. Relax your neck and shoulders. Take a long breath in and slowly breathe out, feeling your feet sink slightly into the floor.

2 Bring your hands in front of you, with your palms facing the floor and your fingertips touching. Extend your arms so that they are as straight as possible, without tensing your shoulders. Slowly raise your arms out to the sides in a wide circle, palms facing outward.

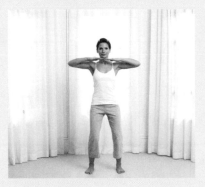

3 Continue the circle upward until your palms are facing the ceiling, with your hands at right-angles to your arms and your fingertips almost touching. Extend your arms away from you, making sure that you haven't lifted your shoulders. Hold for a count of five.

4 Slowly lower your palms in front of you. When your hands are level with your face, rotate your wrists so that your palms face the floor again. Continue to lower your hands until they have reached the starting position in step 2. Repeat steps 2–4 nine times, keeping your actions slow and mindful.

29

afternoon uplifter
energizing

unwind your back and shoulders with gentle swings

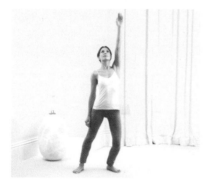 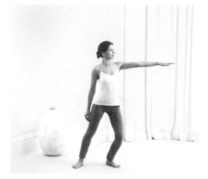

1 Stand with your feet a little wider than hip-width apart and turned out slightly. Shift your weight over your left foot and bend your left knee in line with your toes. Simultaneously, lift your left arm in front of you and stretch it up to the ceiling, moving your head to look up at your hand. Repeat on the right, then alternate sides nine times.

2 Return to the starting position in step 1, but this time stretch your left arm out to the side as you shift your weight and bend your left knee in line with your toes. Turn your head to follow each arm movement and feel yourself reaching out from your waist. Repeat on your right side, then repeat nine times, alternating sides.

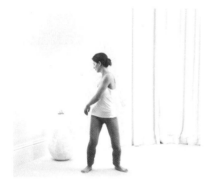

3 Let your arms hang loosely at your sides. Bend your knees and twist your upper body to the right. As you twist, allow your arms to swing gently along with your body. Follow the direction of your body with your head. Keep your lower body stable – don't allow your hips and knees to twist.

4 In a single smooth, continous movement, straighten your knees and swing back to face the front, then bend your knees again as you smoothly twist your upper body to the left. Allow your arms to swing freely, giving your movements momentum. Repeat nine times, alternating sides.

31

1 Stand with your feet shoulder-width apart, your weight evenly distributed over your feet. Bend your knees and feel your spine drop in a long vertical line toward the ground. Tilt your pelvis forward a little to iron out any curve in the lower back. Feel your weight centred in your lower body, while your upper body is light and relaxed. Bring your hands in front of your hips, palms facing inward and fingers loose.

2 Breathe in and, as you breathe out, let your arms float slowly upward. Bend your elbows and keep your palms facing down and toward you. This movement should be slow and relaxed, and your shoulders should not lift at all.

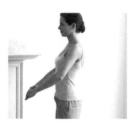

3 Breathe in and continue to raise your arms. Maintain the gentle bend in your elbow. When your hands are level with your face, turn your palms so that you are looking into them. As your arms float further upward, lift your chin to follow the movement of your hands with your head.

4 (right) Now rise up onto your tiptoes, and hold for a count of 10, if you can. Breathe out, lower your heels, bend your knees and return your arms and head to their step-1 position. Repeat the exercise nine times, then place your hands on your abdomen and take 10 slow breaths.

32

evening

de-stress

quietening

instil tranquillity and centredness
with calming chi gung

close
the day
nurturing

treat yourself to a luxurious,
sleep-inducing foot massage

1 Sit on a chair with your back supported. Rest your right foot on your left thigh. Apply a creamy moisturizer all over your right foot. With both hands, stroke your foot from ankle to toes, both on your sole and on the top of your foot.

2 Hold your heel in your left hand and your toes in your right. Circle your foot clockwise around your ankle five times, then five times anticlockwise. Using your right index finger and thumb, stroke your big toe from base to tip, and gently pull the tip to stretch it out. Repeat on each toe in turn, then repeat three times.

3 (*left*) Support the foot with your left hand. Using your right thumb, firmly press into the pad below your big toe. Repeat this pressure on the pad of your next toe, working along to the pad below your little toe. Change hands and, using your left thumb, work in the same way back along your foot pads. Repeat twice.

4 Starting at your heel, press and release with your right thumb, moving along the inner edge of your sole to your big toe. Use your left thumb to repeat this action on the outer edge of your sole, from your heel to your little toe. Repeat the whole exercise on your left foot.

35

bedtime meditation

relaxing

ease into a deep sleep with
a yoga nidra meditation

1 Lie on the floor under a blanket. Become aware of your left foot: heel, toes, sole and the top of your foot. Mentally tell yourself, "My left foot is relaxing. My left foot is relaxed." Bring your awareness to your left leg, and repeat the affirmation: "My left leg is relaxing. My left leg is relaxed." Repeat on your right foot and leg.

2 Become aware of your abdomen, and mentally repeat, "My abdomen is relaxing. My abdomen is relaxed." Feel your back softening against the floor, and mentally repeat, "My back is relaxing. My whole back is relaxed." Focus next on your chest and repeat, "My chest is relaxing. My whole chest is relaxed."

3 Take your attention to your left hand: fingers, palm and the back of your hand. Mentally repeat, "My left hand is relaxing. My left hand is relaxed." Become aware of your arm: wrist, forearm, elbow, upper arm and shoulder. Repeat, "My left arm is relaxing. My left arm is relaxed." Repeat with your right hand and arm.

4 Continue to move your consciousness around your body: to your neck, throat, face (jaw, chin, cheeks, nose, lips, eyes, eyebrows, forehead, ears) and finally your whole head. As you focus on each body part, repeat the relevant affirmation. Feel your body floating, free of tension, your mind relaxed but aware.

1 Try out this stress-relieving technique after a long lie-in on a weekend morning. Sit up in bed with your back supported. Make sure that you are warm and comfortable. Lower your chin to your chest and inhale and exhale slowly four times, feeling any physical tension drain away.

2 Place your hands on either side of your neck, your little fingers just below your ears. Press with your finger pads and release. Move your fingertips toward your spine, and repeat. Work your way inward until your fingertips touch. Move to your hairline. Make small outward 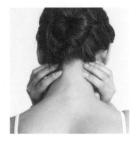 circles with your finger pads along your hairline to your ears. Repeat four times, each time making the circles a little lower down your neck.

3 *(right)* Close your eyes. Place your right hand on your left shoulder and knead along the top of it until you reach your neck. Tilt your head slowly to the left and then to the right. Bring your head upright and repeat the sequence on your right shoulder.

4 Drop your chin to your chest and then raise and lower it slowly, four times. Face straight ahead and roll your shoulders forward four times, then backward four times. Take four long, deep breaths, then let your breath return to its regular pattern and slowly open your eyes.

lazy
weekend
comforting

dispel your tensions after
a tiring week with neck massage

sunday
balance
calming

bring stillness to your
body and mind with yoga

1 This yoga posture is both grounding and uplifting. Stand with your feet hip-width apart, arms by your sides. Close your eyes and focus on your breathing for a moment. Be aware of a sense of inner quiet. Open your eyes and focus your vision on a point about 1m (3ft) in front of you.

2 Raise your left knee and wrap your hands around it. Pull your knee gently up toward your chest, then turn out from your left hip, taking your raised knee out to the side. Place your left foot against your right thigh, as high up your leg as is comfortable. Press the sole of your foot firmly into your thigh.

3 *(left)* Press your knee backward to open up your hip, and bring your hands together in prayer position in front of your breastbone. Slowly move your hands upward until they are above your head, making sure that you keep your shoulders and neck relaxed. Take five long, deep breaths in this position.

4 Release your leg, lower your arms and repeat steps 2–3 with your right leg. Maintaining a visual focus throughout this exercise will aid your balance and concentration. However, if you do lose your balance, simply lower your foot, centre yourself mentally, and raise your foot to your thigh again to continue the exercise.

41

1 Stand straight, feet a little wider than hip-width apart, shoulders relaxed, arms by your sides. Breathe in and draw your navel to your spine. Feel your breath fill your body and lift your arms out to the sides until your hands are at waist level. Breathe out and lower your arms.

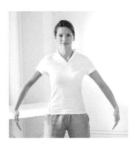

2 Keeping your abdominal muscles drawn in toward your spine, with your next in-breath lift your arms, this time taking them up to shoulder height. Ensure that you initiate the movement from the middle of your back and not from your shoulders. Breathe out and lower your arms.

3 (*right*) Breathe in and lift your arms above your head with your palms facing each other. Breathe out and lower your arms. On your next in-breath, lift your hands to the same position and tilt your head to look into your hands. Feel the stretch reach all the way through your upper body, so that your upper chest also lifts toward the ceiling.

4 Repeat steps 1–3 three times. Finish by returning to the starting pose and checking that you have maintained your posture: back straight, shoulders relaxed, abdominal muscles drawn in toward the spine. You should feel full of oxygen, totally energized and ready for anything!

before a meeting
inspiring
open your heart to fortify your mood

before a night out
steadying

release tension and focus your mind with chi gung

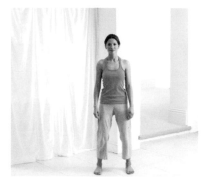

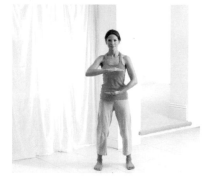

1 Stand with your feet shoulder-width apart, knees slightly bent, arms by your sides. Check that your spine is straight – tilt your pelvis forward a little to flatten your lower back. Your neck and shoulders should be free of tension, loose and relaxed. Take a deep breath in and release it slowly, feeling your feet sink slightly into the floor.

2 Bend your elbows and bring your arms in front of you. Your left hand should be level with your abdomen, your right hand level with your chest, and your palms facing each other, as if you were holding a ball. Lift your left hand up and move your right hand down, so that the backs of your hands face each other.

3 Continue this movement, taking your hands further apart. When your left hand is level with your chin, rotate your palm so that it faces away from you. Continue to push your left hand upward. At the same time, you are lowering your right hand with your palm facing toward the ground.

4 Continue pushing until your arms are completely straight, with your palms at right angles to your wrists. Stretch your arms, then lower them back to the starting position in step 2, but this time with your left arm on top. Push your arms apart to repeat steps 2–4. Repeat eight times, alternating arms in a seamless movement.

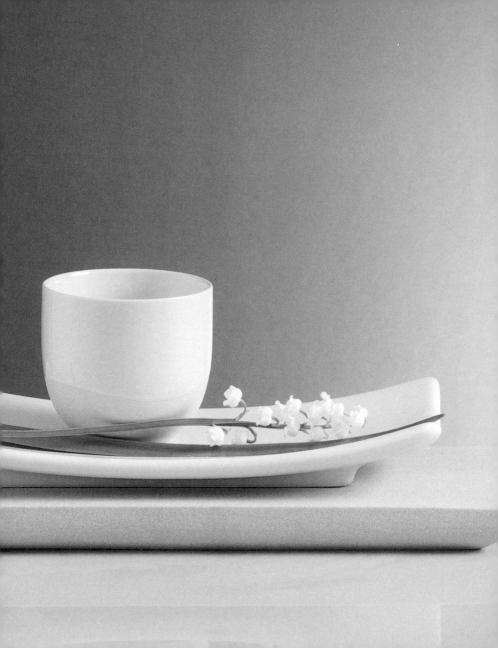

anywhere

The exercises in this chapter will help you to release stress in situations where you might feel it most, such as when you are working or travelling. There are also techniques you can use in places where you are more relaxed, such as in the park or in your own living room. This chapter is your guide to stress busting wherever you are!

in your living room
releasing

loosen your body with a yoga backbend

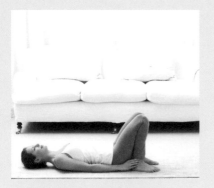 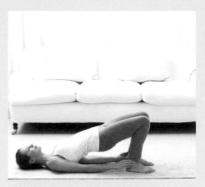

1 Lie on the floor with your arms by your sides and relax for a moment, breathing deeply and letting any tension drain away. Move your heels up close to your buttocks with your feet hip-width apart. Reach your fingers toward your ankles. Grasp the backs of your ankles if you are able to, but be careful not to tense your shoulders.

2 As you breathe in, slowly push upward through your hips to lift them off the floor. Take your hips as high as you can, so that your upper body is in a straight line with your thighs. Hold the pose for a few moments and breathe normally. Make sure your neck, throat and shoulders remain relaxed.

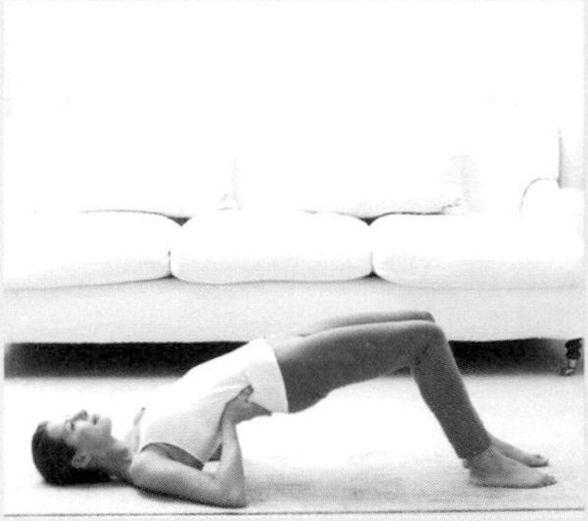

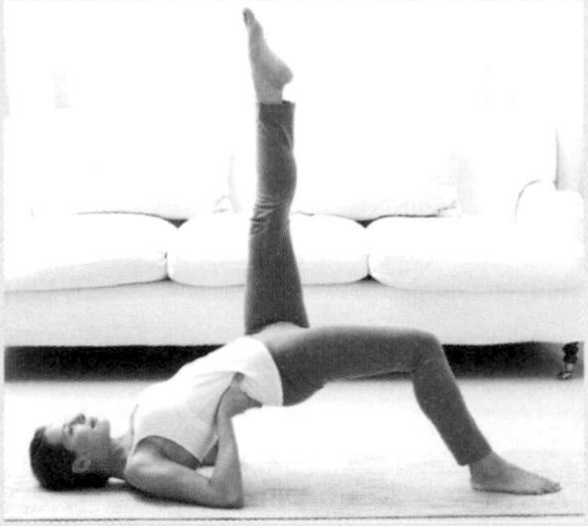

![Two photographs showing bridge pose exercises]

3 Move your hands to support your lower back, fingers pointing toward your heels. Keeping your feet hip-width apart, step them slowly away from your buttocks, as far as you can comfortably reach. Make sure that the soles of your feet are rooted firmly to the ground. Breathe deeply and hold this position for 10 seconds.

4 Breathe in and lift your left leg as high as is comfortable. Straighten your leg and point your toes away from you. Ensure that the rest of your body is in the position from step 3. Breathe out as you lower your left leg, and breathe in to lift your right leg. Breathe out as you lower your body to the floor, straighten your legs and relax.

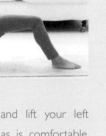

49

1 Position yourself on your sofa however you feel most relaxed. You can sit or lie down as you prefer – just make sure that you are warm and comfortable. Spend a moment focusing on your breath. Imagine yourself opening up as a channel for positive energy.

2 Close your eyes and place your fingers gently over your eyelids. Rest your palms on your cheekbones. Press inward lightly and gently, and focus on being as receptive as possible to external, positive energy. Hold for two minutes, continuing to breathe slowly and deeply.

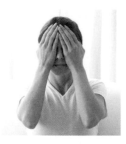

3 *(right)* Place the heels of your hands on your temples. Open up your fingers and wrap them over your head, fingertips pointing toward the crown of your head. Be careful not to cover your ears. Hold this position for two minutes. Visualize positive energy dissolving any anxiety you are feeling, and replacing it with a sense of harmony and inner joy.

4 In both steps 2 and 3, you should feel any lingering tension stored in your facial muscles drain gradually away, softening your face. To conclude the exercise, lower your hands and focus again on your breath for a moment, feeling yourself relaxed and in harmony with the universe.

on your sofa
stabilizing

lift the blues and settle your mind
with a reiki head treatment

in your
bedroom
lightening

**reduce tension-related
headaches**

1 Light an unscented candle and place it on a table. Draw your curtains and dim your lights. Sit comfortably on a chair about 1m (3ft) away from the table. Check that your spine is straight and your shoulders are relaxed. Place your feet flat on the floor and your hands in your lap.

2 Gaze at the candle flame for about 10 seconds without blinking. Then close your eyes and cover them with your palms. Rest the heels of your hands just below your cheekbones and your fingers on your brow. Focus on the flame's image held in your visual memory.

3 (left) Lower your right hand and gaze at the candle with your right eye for 10 seconds. Swap hands, and do the same with your left eye. Remove your right hand and gaze with both eyes for 10 seconds. As you do so, turn your head slowly to the right and then to the left, keeping your eyes focused on the flame.

4 Close your eyes and cover them with your palms for a few moments. Allow your eyes to relax completely. Candle-gazing is highly effective at reducing the frequency of tension-related headaches. With practice, you will be able to extend each period of gazing to 20 or 30 seconds, enhancing the benefits.

53

in your kitchen
invigorating

stretch away upper-body stiffness and tension

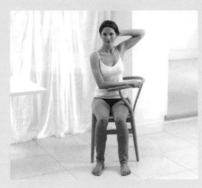 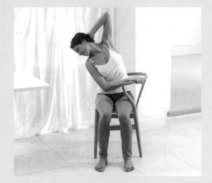

1 Sit sideways on a chair with the left side of your body facing the back of the chair. Place your feet flat on the floor. Cross your right arm in front of your waist and place your right hand on the chair-back. Bring your left hand to the back of your head, making sure that your shoulders stay relaxed.

2 Breathe in and, as you breathe out, turn your head to the right. Lift your elbow toward the ceiling to gently stretch your left side, moving your right shoulder down toward the floor. Breathe in to return to the starting position and repeat five times. Swivel 180 degrees in the chair, and repeat steps 1–2 six times on your right side.

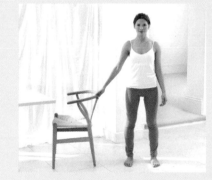

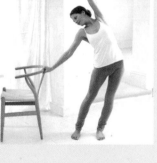

3 Stand with the right side of your body toward the back of the chair, around 45cm (1½ft) away from it. Place your feet hip-width apart, and bring your right hand to the back of the chair. Relax your shoulders, breathe in, then on the out-breath draw your navel gently but firmly toward your spine. Hold it there throughout step 4.

4 Breathe in. As you breathe out, move your left hip away from the chair to stretch the left side of your body. At the same time, bring your left arm out in a wide semi-circle and reach it over your head. Breathe in and return to standing. Repeat five times, then turn so that your left side faces the chair-back and repeat steps 3–4 six times.

1 Lie on the floor on your back, with your legs raised straight up against a wall and your buttocks placed as close to the wall as possible. To release any tension in your face and shoulders, yawn, stretch your arms above your head, then relax your arms down by your sides. Draw your navel gently but firmly toward your spine, and hold it there for the whole of the exercise.

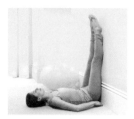

2 Breathe in. As you breathe out, point your toes and, really stretching your legs, slowly draw them apart and down the wall. Take your legs as wide as you comfortably can. If you feel your lower back straining, or if it begins to lift off the floor, bring your legs closer together.

3 *(right)* When you have extended your legs as far as you can, breathe in and, on your next out-breath, flex your feet so that only your heels are touching the wall. Now slowly draw your legs back toward each other. Focus on engaging your inner thigh muscles.

4 Once your legs are back together in their starting position, point your toes again to complete the stretch. Check that your back is still in contact with the floor and that tension has not crept into your lower back and shoulders. Repeat the whole exercise nine times.

in a hotel
restoring

recuperate from a journey with
a blissful Pilates back release

at your desk
opening

climb a ladder of stretches
to soothe tense muscles

1 Sit on a chair with your feet placed a few inches apart and flat on the floor. Rest your hands on your thighs. Draw your navel in toward your spine so that your back straightens. Drop your shoulders. Take three long breaths. Count your inhalation and exhalation, and see if you can make them the same length.

2 Bend your elbows and raise your forearms in line with your upper arms, palms facing outward at shoulder level. Breathe in and stretch your right hand up toward the ceiling, initiating the movement from your shoulder blade. Stretch the whole right side of your body – visualize gaps opening up between your ribs.

3 *(left)* When your arm is fully extended, look up at your hand but don't drop your head back. Instead, feel your spine, neck and head lengthening up toward your fingertips. Breathe out as you bring your chin down and allow your hand to lower back to shoulder height, keeping the lift through your body.

4 Breathe in and repeat steps 2–3 with your left arm. Then alternate arms, as if you were climbing a ladder, until you have completed 10 repetitions on each side. Make sure you take the stretch from your hip all the way through to your fingertips. Breathe slowly and deeply.

1 Sit comfortably and touch the bridge of your nose with your left index finger. Look at your fingertip. Slowly move your finger away from your face, keeping it in focus, until your arm is fully extended. Then draw your finger back to your nose, still maintaining your focus. Repeat twice.

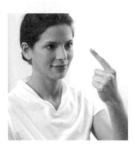

2 Move your index finger to the tip of your nose, and repeat step 1. Slowly extend your arm as before, then move it back, maintaining your visual focus on your finger. You should feel your eye muscles working to accommodate these different focal ranges. Repeat twice.

3 *(right)* Straighten out your left arm at eye level, turning your index finger to point left. Slowly raise your arm, following your finger with your gaze without moving your head. Take your arm as high as you can without your finger disappearing from your visual range. Hold your arm at the highest point for a few seconds, then lower it. Repeat twice.

4 Position your hand at eye level, as it was in step 3. This time move your arm down as low as you can while still focusing on your forefinger and keeping your head still. Repeat twice and then close your eyes and cover them with the palms of your hands to help them to relax.

at your
computer
brightening

banish screen-induced eye strain

1 Stand on the grass in bare feet, with your feet shoulder-width apart. Bend your knees slightly and let your arms hang loosely by your sides. Check that your spine is straight, and tilt your pelvis forward a little to flatten your lower back. Relax your neck and shoulders.

2 Take a long breath in and slowly breathe out, feeling your whole body sink slightly into the ground. Inhale again, deepening the bend in your knees without lifting your heels off the ground. Bring your hands, relaxed and facing inward, level with your solar plexus. Cross your wrists.

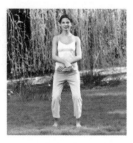

3 *(right)* Breathe in and slowly straighten your knees. At the same time, raise your arms in front of you, keeping your elbows bent and your wrists and hands relaxed. When you have lifted your arms as high as you can without tensing your shoulders, breathe out.

4 Uncross your wrists and lower your arms out to the side until they are level with your shoulders and parallel to the ground. Bend your knees as you do so. Now draw your arms down and in front of you so that they are level with your navel, and cross them at the wrists again. Repeat the whole exercise slowly and rhythmically seven times.

in the park
uplifting

reconnect with nature with
mood-lifting chi gung

on a train
grounding

centre yourself and relax using reflexology pressure points

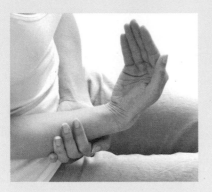 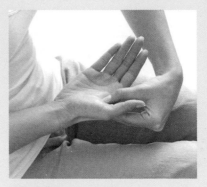

1 Make yourself as comfortable as possible in your seat, with your feet flat on the floor. Check that there is no tension in your neck or shoulders. Bring your right arm in front of you, supporting your right forearm with your left hand. Relax your right hand and rotate it five times clockwise, followed by five times anticlockwise.

2 Using the thumb and index finger of your left hand, press firmly into the gap between the thumb and index finger of your right hand. Make three clockwise circles, then three anticlockwise circles with your left thumb. Move to between your index and middle fingers, and repeat. Work along to your little finger in this way.

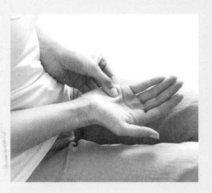 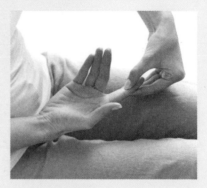

3 Starting at the heel of your right hand, press and release clockwise around the edge of your palm with your left thumb. Pay particular attention to the pads at the base of each finger. Then draw your thumb firmly from the heel of your hand to the base of each finger, working from your little finger to your thumb. Repeat this step five times.

4 Hold the thumb of your right hand near its base with your left thumb and fingers. Draw them up the length of your thumb. As you reach the thumb pad, gently pull to stretch out your thumb. Relax your other fingers. Repeat step 4 with each of your fingers in turn, and then repeat the whole exercise on your left hand.

65

in your car
refreshing

release shoulder and neck tension
and open up your chest

1 Practise this exercise while you are stuck in traffic, or at the end of a stressful drive. Sit up as straight as possible and look straight ahead. Let your arms hang loosely at your sides. Lift your shoulders as high as you can toward your ears, then let them drop heavily. Repeat nine times.

2 *(left)* From this dropped-shoulder position, roll your shoulders forward while keeping your head still and relaxed. Your arms will automatically move so that the backs of your hands are facing forward, but avoid consciously moving your arms.

3 Now lift your shoulders as high as you can toward your ears, keeping your arms relaxed and loose. Continue the circle, rolling your shoulders backward and squeezing your shoulder blades together. Be careful not to over-arch your back.

4 Drop your shoulders to complete the circle. Repeat nine times, rolling your shoulders forward, up and back four times, then backward, up and forward five times, so that you have completed ten repetitions in each direction. If you feel any tension in your neck, drop your head forward to release it.

67

on a plane
reviving

give the little-used muscles of your feet a workout

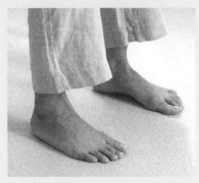 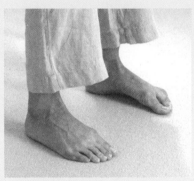

1 Take off your shoes and socks and sit comfortably. Place your feet flat on the floor, hip-width apart, with your knees bent at right angles. Make sure that there is no tension in your upper body and rest your arms and hands loosely in your lap.

2 Draw your toes along the floor toward your heels, so that your insteps lift slightly but your heels stay on the floor. Don't allow your toes to curl under. Hold this position for a few seconds, then relax your feet and straighten your toes. Repeat nine times.

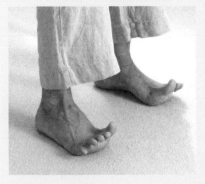 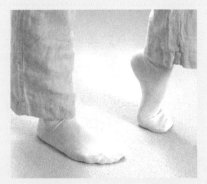

3 Now lift the toes of both your feet upward, while the centre of your sole flattens out against the floor. Stretch your toes as far apart from each other as is comfortable, and hold for a few seconds. Repeat nine times.

4 Put your socks back on and stand up. Find some space, perhaps in the aisle of the plane. Raise your right heel until you are up on your toes, then lower it back to the floor as you begin to lift your left heel in the same way. Repeat nine times, alternating feet in a "walking" motion.

69

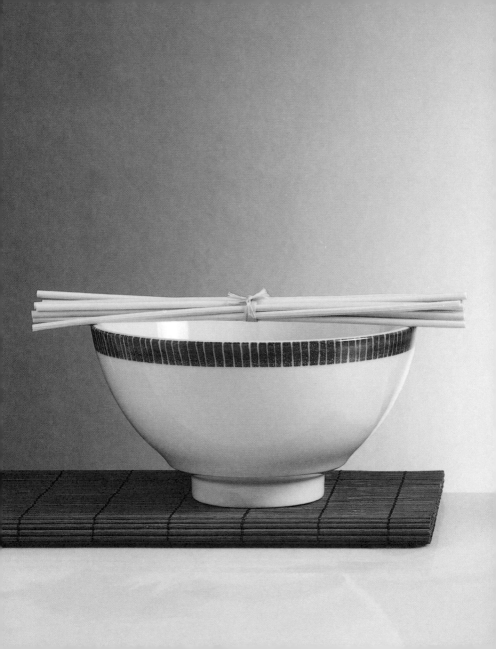

stress-bust your body

Stress tends to affect certain key areas of the body, and when you release these areas, you'll often find that other stress-related physical problems, such as headaches caused by neck or shoulder tension, disappear. So learn to relax and enjoy your body.

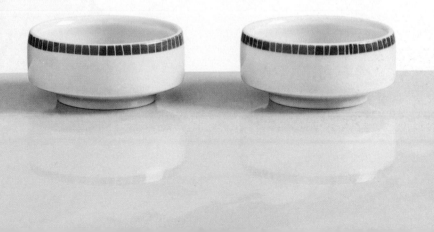

neck loosener
recuperating

use movement and massage to release a stiff neck

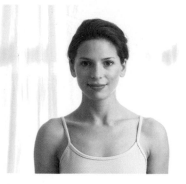 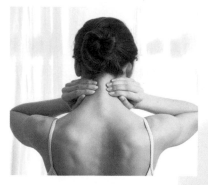

1 Stand with your feet hip-width apart, or sit in a chair with your feet flat on the floor. Relax your shoulders and check that you are not overarching your back (if you are, tuck your tailbone in). Then breathe in, draw your navel toward your spine and hold it there throughout the exercise.

2 Drop your head forward. Place your fingertips horizontally on the back of your neck at your hairline. With your middle-finger pads, make circles outward along your hairline. Repeat five times. Move your fingers to either side of your spine, and make outward circles with your middle-finger pads down your neck. Repeat five times.

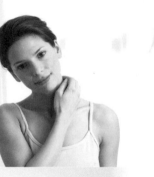

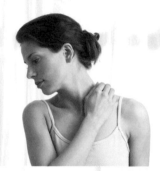

3 Lift your head so that you are facing forward. Tilt your head to the right side and use all your finger pads to massage up the left side of your neck, in the same circular movement you used in step 2. Press firmly to release and loosen your muscles. Repeat, tilting your head to the left side and massaging the right side of your neck.

4 Drop your chin down to your chest and slowly roll your head to the right to look over your right shoulder. Repeat the massage from step 3 with your right hand on the left side of your neck, and then drop your chin to your chest, roll it to the left and repeat the massage on the right side. Alternate from side to side five times.

NECK LOOSENER

headache
reliever
soothing

dissolve headaches with aromatherapy

1 If you regularly suffer from headaches due to stress and overwork, soothe them away with this combination of aromatherapy and relaxation. Begin by creating a "relaxation room". Choose a quiet bedroom, close the curtains, and, if you wish, play some relaxing music.

2 The two essential oils which have particularly therapeutic properties for headaches are lavender and rose. Add eight drops of one of these oils, or four drops of each, to a small bowl of cold water. Soak a large clean cotton handkerchief or a muslin facecloth in the water for a moment.

3 (*left*) Wring out the cloth, lie down and cover yourself with a blanket. Place the soaked cloth across your forehead and close your eyes. Relax for five minutes. Focus on your breathing and release your muscles. If worries appear in your mind, recognize and acknowledge them, and then put them aside to deal with later.

4 If you don't have time or space to lie down, simply moisten your middle fingers with oil and make gentle circles across your forehead, over your temples, behind your ears and across the back of your neck. Unlike the majority of essential oils, lavender and rose are safe to apply directly onto your skin.

75

jaw releaser
alleviating

unlock jaw tension with
a chi gung face massage

1 You may not realize how much tension you are storing in your face. Stress appears in frown lines and strained eyes, but particularly in a clenched, grinding jaw. Stand or sit in front of a mirror, and relax your facial muscles, imagining all the tension flowing out of them.

2 Without straining your neck, tilt your head back so that you are looking up at the ceiling and let your jaw drop open. Push your jaw forward as far as you can and then close it very slowly, in such a way that your bottom teeth touch your top lip. Release your jaw and move your head to look forward. Repeat five times.

3 (left) Looking straight into the mirror, place your hands so that your fingers are resting on your jawline just below your ears. Make small circles toward your ears with your middle fingers, working your way gradually to the centre of your chin, then back to your ears. Keep your jaw relaxed. Repeat five times.

4 Repeat the previous step, but this time use small pinching movements instead of circles. Again, work your way from your ears to the centre of your chin and then back again. Finally, with the finger pads of both hands, pat all over your face creating a gentle, rippling effect.

77

1 This exercise is designed to strengthen your back muscles. When these muscles are strong, they will support all your shoulder and arm movements, meaning that you will no longer strain the shoulders themselves. Stand in a relaxed

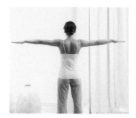

position, feet hip-width apart. Raise your arms to shoulder height, taking care not to lift your shoulders. Turn your palms to face the floor.

2 Breathe in, and as you breathe out, draw your navel in toward your spine. Hold it there for the remainder of the exercise. Now, draw your right arm into your back, moving it backward, downward and inward simultaneously – your right shoulder blade moves toward your spine, while your arm stays fully extended.

3 *(right)* Release your right arm and repeat step 2 with your left arm, then alternate so that you practise step 2 eight times on each side. Then move both arms in at the same time, squeezing your shoulder blades together without arching your back. Release and repeat eight times.

4 To release your back fully, breathe in deeply and wrap your arms around your chest, bringing each hand to the opposite shoulder blade. As you breathe out, drop your chin to your chest. Slowly straighten up your neck, lengthening out your spine. Repeat five times.

shoulder easer
unwinding

relieve painful shoulders and build strength in your back

immunity
booster
fortifying

invigorate a stress-depleted immune
system with hydrotherapy

1 Practise this invigorating technique in your bath tub, or in a large, wide container with shallow sides, such as a washing-up bowl. Dress yourself in warm clothes, but keep your lower legs bare.

2 Fill the tub with very cold water, sufficient to cover your ankles if you were standing in it. You can even throw in some ice cubes if you feel brave enough! The contact of this icy water on your skin will sharply refresh and invigorate your nerves.

3 (left) Step into the water. Walk on the spot, lifting each foot right out of the water in turn. With each step, focus on working right through your foot – carefully place your heel, then your instep, then your toe. Continue treading for 30 seconds, then step out of the water.

4 Dry your feet and ankles, and put on thick, warm socks. Rest for a few minutes, or go straight to bed: cold water treading is an excellent treatment for minor sleep problems and insomnia. When you are used to it, you can use enough water to reach over your calves, and tread for up to three minutes.

IMMUNITY BOOSTER

1 Stand with your feet hip-width apart. Check your posture: your shoulders should be relaxed, your arms hanging loosely by your sides. Draw your navel toward your spine and tuck your tailbone under so that your back is lengthened and the small of your back is not arched.

2 Drop your chin to your chest, feeling the stretch through your neck and upper back. Gradually roll down through your shoulders and upper back, to continue the curve downward. Deepen the curve so that it reaches your lower back and let your arms drop naturally in front of you.

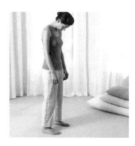

3 *(right)* Breathe deeply and let your entire upper body hang down for a count of five. Keep your legs straight and your weight evenly distributed through your feet. Relax your hands. Sense space opening up between your vertebrae, but don't strain to touch the floor. The weight of your head will automatically stretch your spine.

4 Bend your knees and return slowly to standing, remaining conscious of the stretched-out sensation in your back. Feel your buttock muscles tucking under, anchoring the base of your spine. Unroll your spine vertebra by vertebra. Then let your shoulders drop down naturally and align your neck and head with your spine. Repeat steps 1–4 five times.

back
mobilizer
liberating

let go of back stress
in a simple Pilates roll-down

1 Lie on your back, with your feet resting on a chair so that your legs form a right angle. Place a cushion between your knees. Place your index fingertips and thumbs together to form a diamond shape, and position this over your abdomen. Release any tension from your neck and shoulders. Breathe in and out deeply 10 times, feeling each breath slowly and rhythmically widen your ribs and back.

2 Take another deep breath in and, as you breathe out, draw your navel down toward your spine. Maintain this position, feeling your back lengthen, throughout the rest of the exercise. Gently engage your pelvic floor muscles, then release them. Repeat nine times.

3 (*right*) Breathe in and engage your abdominals to raise your hips off the floor. Lift your spine, vertebra by vertebra, from its base. When you have curled up as far as you can, breathe out and slowly curl down. Take care not to go too far – if your abdominals quiver or you experience any back pain, lower your hips. Repeat nine times.

4 Return to the starting pose and once again breathe in and slowly curl your hips off the floor. This time, raise your arms above your head, placing them on the floor behind you. Breathe out, curl down, lower your arms, and repeat nine times.

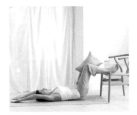

lower-back opener
de-stressing

release your pelvis and lower back with Pilates

body balancer
harmonizing

tone and relax your whole body with a classic yoga sequence

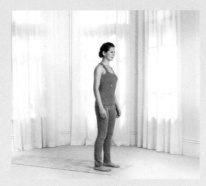 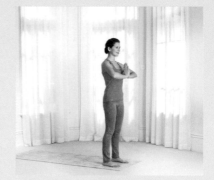

1 This blissfully releasing exercise, known as Salute to the Sun, unifies and balances body and mind. Begin by checking your posture. Stand straight, your feet hip-width apart, your pelvis tilted slightly forward to correct any arch in your lower back and your abdominal muscles engaged and drawn in toward your spine.

2 Breathe in and bring your palms together in prayer position, just in front of your breastbone. Take three more long, deep breaths, and re-focus your attention on your body, noticing and releasing any areas of tension. This concentration on your body will help you to release stress effectively.

3 Breathe in and stretch your arms straight up to the ceiling, keeping the palms of your hands pressed together. Take care not to lift or tense your shoulders. Raise your head to look up into your hands and, if you can do so without any strain in your back, gently bend your upper spine backward.

4 Breathe out and bend forward, keeping your back straight. Fold your body over your legs as far as you can, taking your head toward your knees. Place your hands on your shins, ankles, feet, or on the floor either side of your feet. Breathe in, lift your back and raise your head to look forward, taking care not to strain your neck or shoulders.

87

body balancer

(continued)

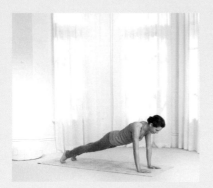

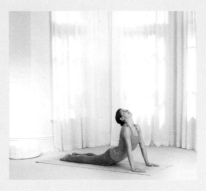

5 Place your hands either side of your feet, bending your knees if you need to. Breathe out and step your feet backward. Lift your abdominals to bring your body to a long, straight plank shape. Align your neck and head with your spine, and straighten your arms and legs. There should be no tension in your shoulders or neck. Breathe in.

6 Breathe out and bend your arms, lowering your knees and chest to the floor, but keeping your abdomen lifted. Breathe in, roll your toes under so that the soles of your feet face the ceiling, and straighten your arms to lift your upper body. If you can, lift your head to look up at the ceiling, but don't strain your neck and shoulders.

7 Breathe out, roll your toes back toward your hands and lift your hips, so that your body forms an inverted V-shape. Relax your head between your arms. Breathe in and step your feet forward between your hands. Place your hands on your shins, ankles, feet, or on the floor either side of your feet, and raise your head to look forward.

8 Breathe out and lower your head toward your knees. Bend your knees, breathe in and slowly raise your upper body. Stretch your arms above your head and bring your palms together. Look into your hands, bending backward if you can, and finally lower your palms in front of your breastbone. Repeat the whole exercise five times.

89

mind

de-stresser

supporting

leave your troubles behind
using autogenic training

1 When you begin autogenic training, practise four sessions in one day: first thing in the morning; mid-morning; mid-afternoon; and finally at bedtime. Continue practising daily until you're familiar with the exercise. To begin your first session, sit on a chair with your feet flat on the floor, or lie down. Close your eyes.

2 Silently repeat the following phrases three times: "My right arm is heavy. My left arm is heavy. Both my arms are heavy. My right leg is heavy. My left leg is heavy. Both my legs are heavy. My arms and legs are heavy." At your second session, add: "My neck and shoulders are heavy. My body breathes me." Repeat three times.

3 At your third session, repeat the phrases in step 2, and add: "My forehead is cool and relaxed. My heartbeat is calm and regular." Repeat three times. For your fourth session, repeat all of the above phrases and then add: "My mind is calm and serene." Repeat three times.

4 As you add each phrase, focus your mind on the area you are naming. Feel the sensation of each body-part relaxing, and take your awareness within to sense your heartbeat. Once you are used to this technique, you can use it for instant calm in any stressful situation.

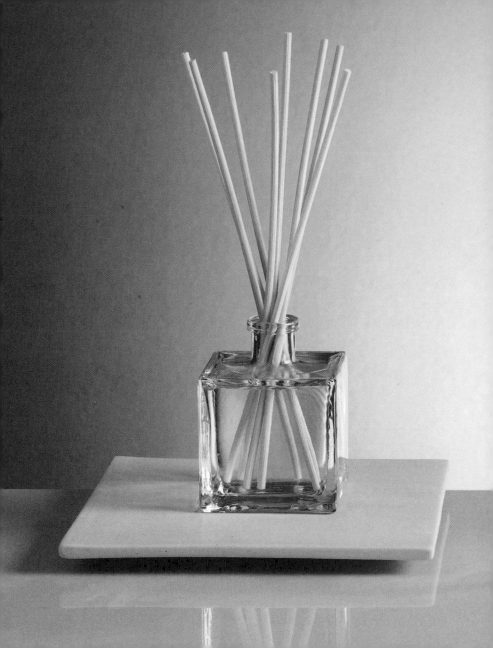

mood
enhancers

These exercises will lift your mood when stress depletes your spirits.

Relaxation techniques, concentration, focusing on your breathing and

simply laughing away tension can all change your state of mind and

leave you feeling much more cheerful, composed and in control.

1 Stand with your feet hip-width apart facing a heavy table or sideboard at around hip-height. Position yourself about 1m (3ft) away from the table and bend your upper body forward. Your fingers should rest on the surface; move your feet forward or backward as necessary.

2 Stand with your navel drawn in toward your spine, and check that there is no tension in your body. Lift and drop your shoulders, position your head so that it feels as if it is being drawn up to the ceiling by an invisible string, and take three slow, deep breaths.

3 (*right*) Bend from your hips, reaching forward so that your fingers rest on the table. Lengthen out your spine to make it as flat as the table-top. Move your tailbone backward to increase the stretch – you may need to move your feet. Drop your head down, releasing any tension in your neck or shoulders. Hold for one minute, breathing deeply.

4 Raise your head to level with your arms. Keeping your back flat and your head and neck in line with your spine, slowly bend your knees, keeping your heels on the floor. Straighten your legs and then slowly bend your knees again, repeating 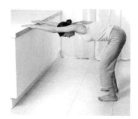 this movement in a constant motion three times. Finally roll up slowly to standing. Feel your spine "stack up", vertebra by vertebra.

upper-body
reviver
rejuvenating

free your body from hips to shoulders

heart
lightener
exhilarating

recover your optimism with this
wonderful reiki technique

1 Sit comfortably on a chair, or cross-legged on the floor with your back against a wall. Stretch your arms up over your head, bring them slowly down to your sides and let them drop. Yawn widely and feel yourself relax. Close your eyes.

2 Allow your awareness to move around your body, mentally checking for any areas of tension and releasing them. Now focus on your breath, feeling the rise and fall of your abdomen. Breathe deeply for one minute, feeling totally relaxed.

3 *(left)* Start to laugh, feeling the corners of your mouth lift and letting the movement spread to your whole body, including your abdomen. Even if it seems like a false laugh at first, just let the physical feeling of laughter take over your body.

4 Start to enjoy the laughter – notice how it affects your body, how it lifts your emotions. Laugh for a full minute. Then compose yourself and examine the state of both body and mind. You may be surprised at how uplifted you now feel.

97

spirit lifter enhancing

allieviate anxiety or depression with a simple chi gung exercise

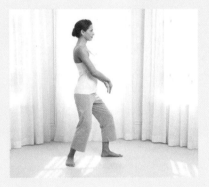 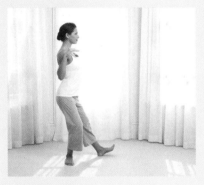

1 Stand with your left foot about 50cm (1½ft) in front of your right one. Turn the toes of your right foot out to the side, and point your left foot forward. Bend your knees deeply, without lifting your heels and distribute your weight evenly between your feet. Cross your wrists in front of you level with your navel, palms facing inward.

2 Breathe in and take your weight backward over your right foot. Bend your right knee more – you'll find your left knee will automatically straighten. Raise the toes of your left foot. Bend your elbows, drawing back your forearms so that they move toward your body. Relax your hands level with your shoulders, palms facing outward.

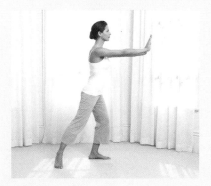

3 Breathe out as you take the weight back on to your left foot and lift up your right heel, keeping your toes on the ground. At the same time, push your hands forward in a smooth motion, palms flat and facing outward. Don't allow this movement to cause tension in your shoulders or neck.

4 Breathe in and transfer your weight backward once again so that it is over your right foot. Draw your arms back, bending your elbows, so that you return to the position in step 2. Alternate between steps 3 and 4 nine times, then swap feet so that your right foot is in front. Repeat the whole exercise 10 times.

99

breath
invigorator
clearing

sweep worries from your mind
with dynamic breathing

1 Sit on the floor or, if you prefer, on a chair with your feet flat on the floor. Your spine should be long and straight, your shoulders relaxed and your hands placed loosely on your thighs. Close your eyes and focus on your breath, feeling it rise and fall in your chest and abdomen.

2 Take a deep breath in, and visualize the passage of your breath through your body, as it brings oxygen through your lungs and into your bloodstream, energizing every cell. Breathe out and visualize tiredness, anxiety and any other negative feelings flowing out of your body.

3 *(left)* Inhale deeply through your nose, and breathe out through your mouth. As you do so, contract your abdominal muscles sharply and continuously so that you make repeated exhalations with a "ha" sound. Make your out-breath last for 10 of these smaller exhalations.

4 Take three normal breaths, then place one hand on your chest and the other on your abdomen, and repeat step 3. The position of your hands will help you really feel the movement of breath in and out of your body. Repeat step 3 five times, gradually building up to 20 mini-exhalations on each out-breath.

1 Lie on your back with your knees raised and arms stretched out at shoulder level. Soften your shoulders and neck. Place a tennis ball between your knees and raise your feet in the air so that your lower legs are at right angles to your thighs.

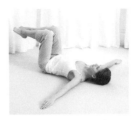

2 Breathe in and, as you breathe out, draw your navel gently but firmly toward your spine. Hold it there throughout the remainder of the exercise. Let your lower back relax against the floor. Check that this does not cause any tension in your neck and shoulders.

3 (*right*) Breathe in and, as you breathe out, slowly lower your knees down to your left toward the floor, while you turn your head to the right. Allow your feet to rest on the floor for support. Don't allow your right shoulder to lift or tense, and keep your neck relaxed. Feel a strong diagonal stretch across your body and hold for a count of five.

4 Breathe in and, as you breathe out, raise your knees and move your head back to the centre. Repeat on the right side, turning your head to the left. Make sure that your abdominal muscles are doing the work and that your lower back is not arching. Practise the whole exercise ten times on each side, moving as slowly as you can.

MOOD ENHANCERS

back booster
freeing

twist away tension to elevate your mood

body stimulator revitalizing

refresh your body and mind in invigorating yoga poses

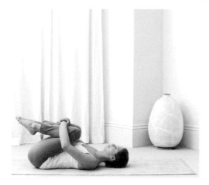

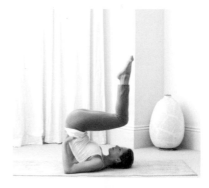

1 Lie flat on the floor with your arms by your sides. Check that there is no tension in your neck or shoulders and relax your whole body. Breathe in and, as you breathe out, bend your knees up to your chest and hug them inward, to help you to correct any over-arching in your lower back.

2 Release your legs and, on your next out-breath, raise your hips off the floor. Bring your legs over your head, and use your hands to support your lower back. Continue to raise the rest of your back off the floor.

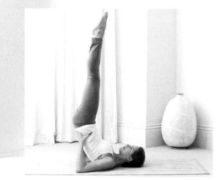

3 When your back is as vertical as you can manage, straighten your legs and point your toes. As your body rises above your head, it will press your chin toward your chest, stimulating your thyroid gland. Engage your abdominal muscles and hold this position for up to one minute, breathing deeply.

4 If you are comfortable in this position, on an out-breath allow your feet to drop gently behind your head. Be careful to keep your back extended. Touch the floor with your toes, then inhale to return to the vertical position from step 3. Slowly roll your back down onto the floor.

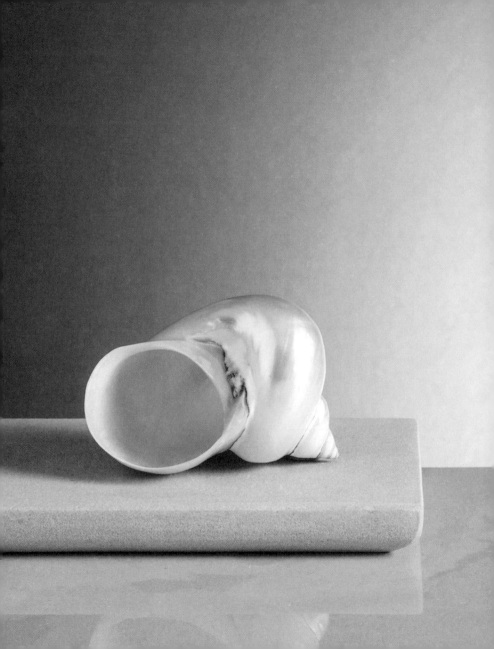

practising together

Working with a partner has both practical and emotional benefits. You can help each other move into deep stretches, and bring a new level of enjoyment to massage and reiki treatments. Be sensitive to your partner – check that levels of stretch and pressure are appropriate for them, and work together to maintain a tranquil atmosphere.

energy balancer
reassuring

de-stress your partner with soothing reiki

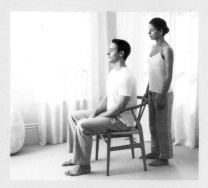 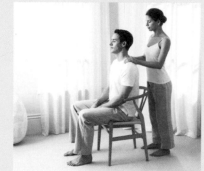

1 Ask your partner to sit comfortably on a chair, with their feet flat on the floor, their spine straight and relaxed, and their eyes closed. Stand behind the chair with your eyes closed. Feel totally relaxed. Visualize healing energy pouring into your body and circulating around it. You will channel this energy into your partner.

2 Make the first physical contact by laying your hands gently on your partner's shoulders. Hold this position for two to three breaths. Continue to imagine the positive energy flowing into your body, and passing through your hands into your partner's body.

108

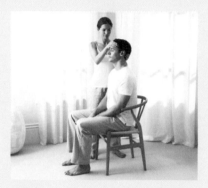

3 Carefully lay one hand on each side of your partner's head. Stay for two to three breaths. Make sure that your touch is gentle and light, and keep your fingers together. Remove your hands and stand on your partner's right. Place your right hand on their forehead and your left hand on the nape of their neck. Hold for two or three breaths.

4 Place your left hand at the top of your partner's spine and your right hand just below their neck. Your hands should be flat and at right angles to your partner's spine. Hold for two to three breaths. Place your right hand on your partner's upper chest and your left hand between their shoulder blades. Hold for two to three breaths.

109

energy balancer

(continued)

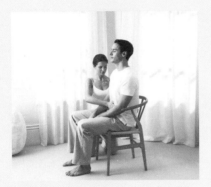

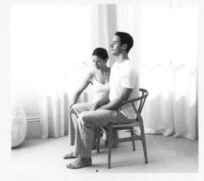

5 Kneel down beside your partner. Place your right hand over their solar plexus, just beneath their rib-cage, and your left hand on their back, level with your right hand. Hold for two to three breaths. Move your right hand down to your partner's navel, again bringing your left hand level on their back. Stay here for two to three breaths.

6 Change the position of your left hand so that your fingers point downward and your palm covers your partner's lower spine. Place your right hand on your partner's right knee, cupping their knee-cap. Hold for two to three breaths. Move to your partner's left side and repeat, using your opposite hands for your partner's back and knee.

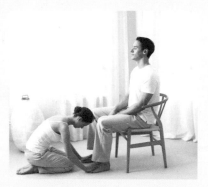

7 Kneel down in front of your partner. Place your hands on their feet, with the heels of your hands resting on their toes, your palms covering the tops of their feet and your fingers reaching up toward their ankles. Stay here for two to three breaths.

8 Return to step 5, placing your right hand over your partner's solar plexus and your left hand on their back. Stay for two to three breaths. Return to step 3, placing your hands either side of your partner's head. Stay for two to three breaths, then remove your hands. Ask your partner to rest for a few breaths, with their eyes closed.

111

1 Ask your partner to kneel on the floor sitting on their heels. Sit or kneel behind them. You should both keep your spines long and straight and your shoulders loose so that your bodies feel relaxed. Bring your hands to your partner's shoulders to check that they are relaxed.

2 Ask your partner to inhale and lift their hands above their head, then exhale, drop their arms to the floor and bend forward from their hips. They should place their forehead on the floor and their arms relaxed by their sides. Their toes should be tucked under, facing the ceiling.

3 Bring your thumbs to either side of the base of your partner's spine. Press in with your thumbs and make gentle circles away from their spine, all the way up to their neck. Kneel on your partner's left side. Bring your left hand to their left

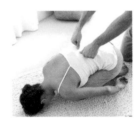

shoulder, and your right hand to their right hip. Gently push your hands apart to create a diagonal stretch. Move to your partner's right side and repeat, using opposite hands for the opposite shoulder and hip.

4 (*right*) Place your right hand between your partner's shoulder blades, and your left hand on the base of their spine. Press down onto the heels of your hands and move them apart to stretch your partner's back. If you can, gently push your partner's buttocks onto their heels.

tension
reliever
centering

unravel your partner's tensions
in this deeply relaxing yoga pose

back extender
lengthening

banish your worries with a double-strength stretch

1 Sit on the floor facing each other with your spines as straight as possible and your legs wide apart. Bring the soles of your feet against your partner's. Both stretch out your arms, and hold each other's hands. You may need to lean forward – if you do, bend from your hips, keeping your backs absolutely straight.

2 (*left*) Reach your fingers down each other's arms so that you are holding wrists. Breathe in, and, as you breathe out, lean back slowly with a straight back, stretching your partner forward with a flat back. Take care not to strain your partner's hips, knees or back. If you can, hold the position for a count of ten.

3 Use your abdominals to bring yourself back up to centre, as your partner does the same. Now your partner leans back, so that you reverse roles and it is your turn to stretch forward. It is important that you keep your back flat throughout the stretch, so only go as far as is comfortable. If you can, hold for a count of ten.

4 Continue reversing roles until you have both stretched forward five times, reaching a little further forward each time but keeping your backs straight. If you are both flexible, you may find that you need to hold further up your partner's arms to achieve a satisfying stretch.

1 Ask your partner to lie down on the floor with their head on a pillow and their eyes closed. Cover their whole body from the neck down with a blanket – this will keep them warm as their temperature drops during relaxation. Kneel comfortably behind your partner's head.

2 Begin by running your hands through your partner's hair several times, tracing your fingers over their scalp and working from the hairline backward. Then, gently take a handful of hair and pull lightly. Repeat all over your partner's head.

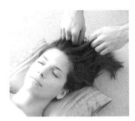

3 Press with your thumbs from the centre of their forehead along the mid-line of their scalp to the back of their head. Repeat twice, each time starting slightly lower on the forehead. Massage your partner's ears between your index fingers and thumbs, from the lobes round to the tops. Repeat twice, then cover their ears briefly with your palms. Press along your partner's eyebrows with your index finger pads.

4 (*right*) With your thumbs, press gently just below their nose, then press outward in a line under the cheekbones toward the ears. Beginning just below their lips, repeat, following the same line. Then, starting from the centre of the chin, gently pinch their jawline between your index finger and thumb, all the way out to just below their ears.

mind
restorer
regenerating

induce profound relaxation with
a shiatsu massage

body relaxer
softening

unknot strain in your partner's back with a soothing massage

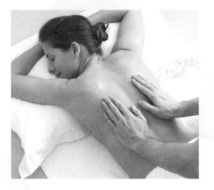

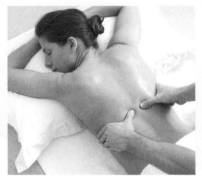

1 Ask your partner to undress to the waist and lie face-down on the floor with their head turned to one side on a pillow, and hands above their head. Cover their body with a towel, from the base of their spine to their feet. Warm some massage oil in your palms, place your hands on your partner's shoulders and stroke down their back.

2 Place your thumbs either side of the base of their spine, and work up to their shoulders making little circles toward the sides of their body. Knead their shoulder muscles with your fingers and then stroke down their back. Repeat three times. After the third time kneading, rhythmically squeeze all over the shoulder area, alternating hands.

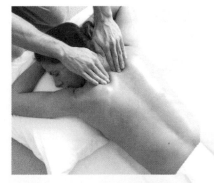 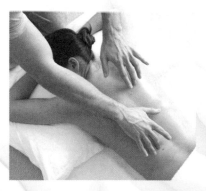

3 Move so that you are kneeling at the top of your partner's head. Using both your hands, carefully squeeze, knead, and make small circles around their neck area and the top of their shoulders. Using firm strokes, try to release any knots. Check with your partner that the level of pressure you are applying is comfortable for them.

4 Stroke alternate hands from the base of your partner's spine up to their neck. As one hand reaches your partner's neck, start the stroke with your other hand. Lighten your touch with each repetition until you are gently brushing your partner's back with your middle fingertips. Cover your partner with the towel and leave them to relax.

1 (*right*) Sit back-to-back on the floor, making sure your shoulders are relaxed. Bring the soles of your feet together in front of you, and let your knees relax out to the sides. The closer your soles are to your body, the harder your hips will need to work, so stay at a level that is comfortable for you. Hold your ankles for support.

2 Both of you breathe in deeply through your noses, feeling the breath fill your bodies, so that your ribs widen and your abdomens rise. Continue focusing on your breath for one to two minutes. On an out-breath, both draw your navels toward your spine. Keep your abdominal muscles engaged in this way for the remainder of the exercise.

3 Breathe out and lean forward slightly, feeling your partner's weight sink into your back. Keep your heads and necks in line with your spines. Breathe in as you lean backward, and your partner leans forward. Repeat three times.

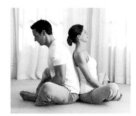

4 Return to the upright position. Check that your shoulders are down and your abdominal muscles are still engaged. Stay in this position for a further minute, breathing deeply and letting your knees fall as far as possible toward the floor. Then bring your knees together and relax.

core
strengthener
sustaining

improve your posture and boost your inner confidence

torso stretcher activating

stretch out and release your partner's torso muscles

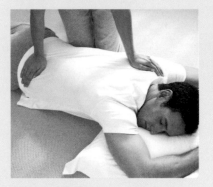 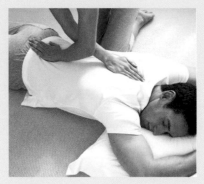

1 Ask your partner to lie on the floor, with their head turned to one side and their arms and head resting on a pillow. Kneel on their left side. Place your left hand on their left shoulder, and your right hand on their right hip. Push your hands apart. Hold for one minute, then repeat the stretch on their opposite shoulder and hip.

2 Now place the heel of your left hand in the middle of your partner's lower back, with your fingers pointing toward their legs. Place the heel of your right hand in between your partner's shoulder blades, pointing your fingers toward their head. Press down to stretch out your partner's spine. Hold the stretch for one minute.

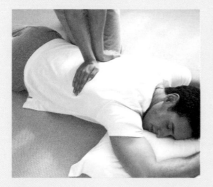

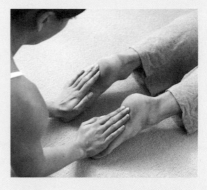

3 Place the heels of your hands on your partner's shoulder blades, wrapping your fingers over the sides of their body. Press down with as much weight as is comfortable for your partner. Inch your way down the sides of your partner's spine all the way to the base, pressing as you go. Continue down the length of their legs.

4 Now place your hands on your partner's feet, with the heels of your hands resting on the backs of their toes and your fingers pointing toward the heels. Press gently with your hands up along the soles of the feet, then cover your partner with a blanket and leave them to rest for a few minutes.

123

everyday sequences

When you have a little more time, why not practise a longer stress-busting sequence? The half-hour menus below focus on a single discipline, while the one hour sequences combine several. Practise these exercises in any suitable location.

index

acknowledgments

publisher's acknowledgments

Duncan Baird Publishers would like to thank the models Serina Curruthers and Stephen Bracken, hair and make-up artist Tinks Reding, and photographer's assistant Adam Giles.